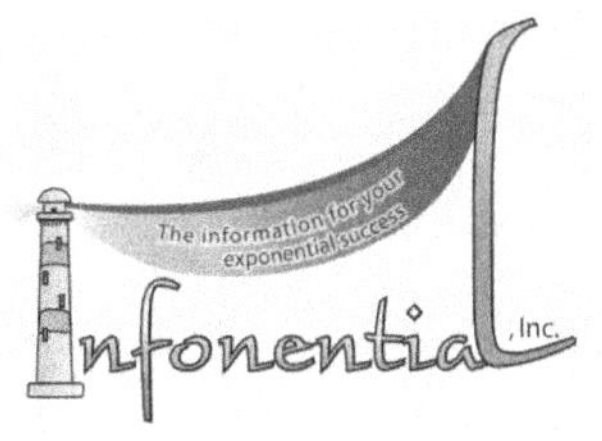

Biotechnology Flashcard Quicklet

Flashcards in a Book for Biotech Students

Paul Sanghera, Ph.D.

Biotechnology Flashcard Quicklet: Flashcards in a Book for Biotechnology Students

Published by
Infonential, Inc.
A California Corporation.
http://www.infonentialinc.com
email: info@infonentialinc.com

ISBN-10: 0-9791797-6-9
ISBN-13: 978-0-9791797-6-1

This publication is designed to provide accurate and authoritative information on the covered subject matter. It can be used by the students of biotechnology in conjunction with a textbook for a quick review of the subject matter. However, it is sold with the understanding that the publisher is not engaged in offering technical, legal, or other professional service. If such assistance is required, the service of a competent professional should be sought.

Warning and Disclaimer
The information published in this book has been obtained by Infonential, Inc. from sources believed to be reliable. We have made our best effort to make this material as comprehensive within the scope of this book and as accurate as possible. However, because of possible errors such as human, mechanical, or technical, the publisher and the author does not guarantee the accuracy, adequacy, or completeness of any information and are not responsible for any errors or omissions and the results obtained from such information.

To
The Teachers of Biotechnology
Mousa Ghanma, Laurie Issel-Tarver, Nita Sharma
And many others
For their invaluable contributions
To the field

Table of Contents

The Quicklet Book Series

The purpose of a *quicklet* book is to present the required information on a subject within a well defined scope by focusing on the customer needs.

The lack of information is the problem of the past ages. The problem of the current age, the information age, is that we have too much information and too little time to absorb it. We are being bombarded with all kinds of needed and (mostly) unneeded information from all sides. This situation has created the need for information products that contain well defined, precise, to the point, quick, and "just what the customer needs" information. The *Quicklet Book Series* is a response to this market need. In other words, a *quicklet* is based on the philosophy that in this fast paced information age, nobody has the time to prowl through web pages or struggle with a 700 pages long book to find just that little piece of needed information.

Bottom line: A *quicklet* offers maximum learning in minimum time. No fluff, just the nuggets of the needed information presented in an easy to understand format.

About the Author

Dr. Paul Sanghera, an educator, scientist, technologist, and an entrepreneur, has a diverse background in all the fields on which biotechnology is based including physics, chemistry, biology, computer science, and math. He holds a Master degree in Computer Science from Cornell University, a Ph.D. in Physics from Carleton University, and a B.Sc. with triple major: physics, chemistry, and math. He has taught science and technology courses all across the world including San Jose State University and Brooks College. Dr. Sanghera has been involved in educational programs and research projects in biotechnology. He has authored and co-authored more than 100 research papers published in well reputed European and American research journals.

As a technology manager, Dr. Sanghera has been at the ground floor of several technology startups. He is the author of several best selling books in the fields of science, technology, and project management. He lives in Silicon Valley, California, where he currently serves as Assistant Professor at California Institute of Nanotechnology.

About This Book

Dr. Sanghera offers a taste of the discipline of biotechnology by presenting more than 325 flashcards in this easily portable book. Primarily designed to be used with your textbook, this book is also a quick introduction to (or overview of) biotechnology. Although the book is self contained within its scope, it assumes that you have already studied the material from a textbook on biotechnology, and use this book as a quick review and reference.

Special features:

- Most of the essential concepts, terms, formulae, and processes are covered.

- The depth and style of the coverage makes these flashcards indexes into your memory so that if you go through these flash cards after reading a textbook, it's almost equivalent to going through the textbook once again, only in much less time.

- The flashcards are largely self-contained and no reference to any other book is made.

How to use this book: Read the front of a page and answer it. Then look at the back of the page to check if your answer was correct.

Welcome to the discipline of biotechnology.

Enjoy.

Q1

What is science?

Q2

In which way science is a process?

A1

Science is the body of knowledge about the natural world organized in a rational and verifiable way. The word *science* has its origin in a Latin word that means "to know". Science is organized into different fields or branches such as physics and chemistry. Mathematics (math in short) is considered to be the language of science, as it is used to express science, for example, in formulas.

A2

Science is a way of knowing. It involves discovery, which can use a process of inductive reasoning. It can also use hypothesis testing, which is also a process.

Q3

What is biology?

Q4

What are organisms and microorganisms?

A3

Biology is the branch of science that studies life. The word biology has a Greek origin: *bio* means life and *logos* means knowledge. Biology is also referred to as biological sciences because it has a broad spectrum of fields including botany (study of plants), zoology (study of animas), cellular biology (study of basic building blocks of life), microbiology (study of microorganisms), and ecology (study of interrelations among organisms).

A4

microorganism An organism that is too small to be seen by human eye

organism A living adaptive system of organs with organs interacting in such a way that they work as a single whole.

organ A collection of tissues that perform a set of functions.

tissue A collection of interconnected cells within an organism with each cell performing a similar function.

cell The smallest metabolically functional unit of life largely made of protein and DNA.

adaptive system A system capable of learning from experience, and changing accordingly.

Q5

Biology is based on which two branches of science?

Q6

What is chemistry?

A5

Physics and chemistry

The foundations of biology are based on physics and chemistry. In other words, biology applies the laws of physics and chemistry to living things.

A6

Chemistry is the branch of science that deals with the composition, properties, and interactions (reactions) of matter especially at the atomic and molecular levels.

Q7

What is biochemistry?

Q8

What is biotechnology?

A7

The study of the fundamental chemistry of living things, that is, organisms

A8

Any technology that uses biological systems, living organisms, or parts of living organisms to make or modify products, processes, or applications for specific uses.

Q9

What are the characteristics of living things?

Q10

What is the complexity of organization in organisms?

A9

- **Complexity of organization**
- **Ecology**
- **Evolution**
- **Growth**
- **Metabolism**
- **Reprodction**
- **Responsiveness**

A10

Complexity of organization refers to the complex and sophisticated structure of organisms. For example, an organism is composed of organs, which are composed of tissues. A tissue in turn is composed of cells with each cell performing a similar function. Each cell is composed of molecules.

Q11

What is ecology?

Q12

What is evolution?

A11

Ecology is the study of releationships among different organisms and the realtionships of organisms with their environment.

A12

Evolution may be defined as a change in the genetic composition of a genetic population from generation to generation as a result of processes such as natural selection and mutation. This continuous change ultimately results in the development of new species.

Q13

What is the growth chaarctersitic of a living organism?

Q14

What is metabolism?

A13

The ability to grow; this is the ability of an organism to take in the appropriate material from its environment and convert it into a part of its own structure. Eating and digesting food is an example.

A14

The set of all biochemical processes (chemical reactions) occurring in a living cell of an orgnaism. These processes enable cells to maintain their structure, grow, reproduce, and respond to their environemnt. In this way, metabolism provides the basis of life. It involves two steps: converting the consumed material into energy, called catabolism, and using that energy to build cell commpnents, called anabolism.

Q15

What is reproduction?

Q16

What are the two types of reproduction?

A15

A fundamental feature of life that enables organisms to produce new organisms. All organisms exist as a result of reproduction.

A16

Sexual Two individual organisms (parents) participate in producing the new individual. Humans reproduce through sexual reproduction.

Asexual An individual (one parent) can reproduce without the participation of another individual. Most plants have the ability for asexual reproduction.

Science of Biotechnology

Q17

What is responsiveness?

Q18

What is a scientific method?

A17

The ability of living things to respond to the external stimuli (the stimuli in the external environment). Examples of stimuli are light, sound, heat, and contact. Humans use five senses (seeing, hearing, smell, taste, and touch) to detect the stimuli.

A18

A process to obtain scientific knowledge. It has the following three general steps:

1. Observe a phenomenon and state the problem

2. Formulate hypothesis that explains observation. Make predictions based on the hypothesis

3. Test the hypothesis and predictions through experiments

Q19

What is the difference between a theory and a law?

Q20

What is physics?

A19

A hypothesis is a logical and verifiable explanation of a phenonmenon or observations that makes some predictions. A hypothesis that passes the experimental tests is usually called a theory. A well tested and widely accepted theory is usually accepted as a law among the scientific community.

A20

Physics is that branch (or discipline) of science that deals with understanding the universe and the systems in the universe in terms of fundamental constituents of matter (such as atoms, electrons, and quarks) and the interactions between those constituents.

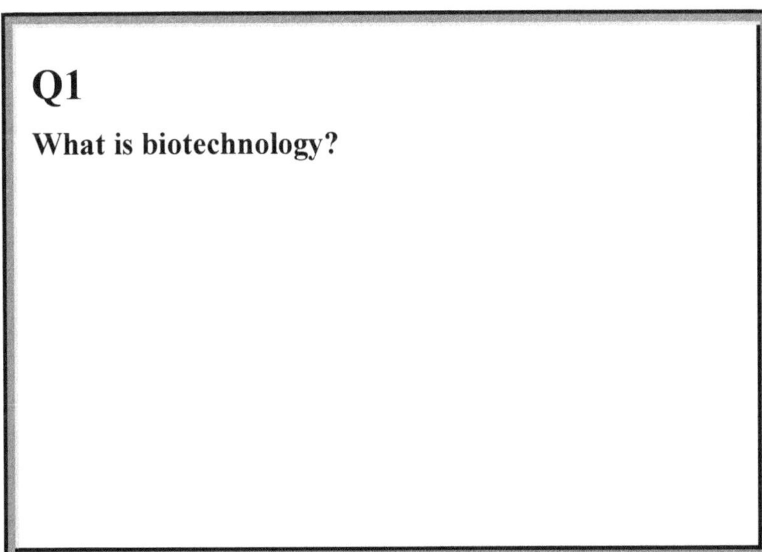

Q2

Researchers in biotechnology use knowledge, tools, techniques, and processes from which fields?

A1

According to the United Nations Convention on Biological Diversity:

"Biotechnology means any technological application that uses biological systems, living organisms, or derivatives thereof, to make or modify products or processes for specific use."

Equivalently, biotechnology can also be defined as study and manipulation of living organisms or their components such as organs, tissues, cells, and molecules, for different purposes such as performing research and developing products and applications.

A2

- ◆ **Biology**
- ◆ **Chemistry**
- ◆ **Computer science**
- ◆ **Physics**

Q3

List some techniques and practices of biotechnology.

Q4

What is cloning?

A3

- ♦ **Cloning**
- ♦ **Fermentation**
- ♦ **Recombinant DNA**

A4

The technique (or process) to generate a genetically identical copy of an organism, cell, or a DNA fragment (molecule).

For example, human cloning refers to creating a new human who will be genetically identical copy of a living or a dead human.

Dolly the sheep (07/05/1996 – 02/14/2003) was the first mammal that was cloned from an adult cell at Roslin Institute in Scotland. Her birth was announced in February 1997.

Q5

What is fermentation?

Q6

What is recombinant DNA technique?

A5

A technique or process to create energy in a cell by converting sugar into lactic acid or ethanol. Sugars are the common substrate (initial substance or reactants) of fermentation.

A common example:

Yeast is used as a catalyst to carry out fermentation in order to produce ethanol in alcoholic drinks such as beer or wine.

A6

A technique for splitting and recombining the DNA molecules. A recombinant DNA molecule is a DNA molecule that contains DNA from at least two different sources.

This ability to cut and paste DNA enables biotechnology companies to develop a wide variety of products and applications. Human insulin is an example.

 Introduction to Biotechnology

Q7

What is human insulin?

Q8

What is diabetes?

A7

A protein (polypeptide hormone) that regulates the metabolism by faciliatating uptake of sugar from blood into cells. Genetically engineered insulins are used for the treatment of diabetes.

A8

A disorder that affects the uptake of sugar from blood into cells resulting in high sugar in the blood

Q9

What are antibiotics?

Q10

What is DNA?

A9

A chemical substance produced by a few species of bacteria or fungi that kills some other microrganisms. The first antibiotic product developed as medicine was penicillin to treat infections.

A10

Deoxyribonucleic acid; a nucleic acid that contains the genetic information used to produce proteins.

Q11

What is the genome of an organism?

Q12

What is the Human Genome Project?

A11

An entire set of genetic material from a single cell of the organism

A12

A project that involved international collaboration and was set up to identify all the genes and their sequence in the human genome.

 Introduction to Biotechnology

Q13

What are the major categories of products that most of the biotechnology companies develop?

Q14

What kinds of jobs are available in biotechnology?

A13

- Agricultural
- Industrial
- Pharmaceutical
- Research and production tools

A14

- Quality assurance
- Manufacturing
- Project management
- Lab technician
- Research and development
- Technical writing

Q15

What is culture in biology?

Q16

What is genetics?

A15

A method of growing a microbiological organism

A16

The study of genes that includes the issues such as how genes are inherited and expressed. A gene is a segment of DNA that contains the genetic information.

 Introduction to Biotechnology

Q17

What is t-PA?

Q18

Inserting the missing piece of gene (code) into a patient's cells is part of a treatment called:

A17

Tissue plasminogen activator; an enzyme that can be used to clear blocked blood vessels immediately after a heart attack by dissolving, that is, breaking down blood clots.

Human body produces t-PA in very small amounts. Biotechnologists have developed genetical enginering techniques to produce t-PA by using Chinese hamster ovary (CHO) cells.

A18

Gene therapy

Q1

What is biomanufacturing?

Q2

What is pharmaceutical industry?

A1

The industry that focuses on producing the products created by using biotechnology such as proteins

A2

The industry focused on producing drugs used for medical purposes. Some of these drugs may be produced by using biotechnology. So, there is a relationship between biomanufacturing and pharmaceutical industry. However, biomanufacutring is not limited to creating pharmaceutical products; it also creates products in other application areas such as agriculture.

Q3

What are the raw materials for biomanufacturing?

Q4

What is cytology?

A3

Living organisms and their components such as organs, tissues, cells, protein, DNA, and other molecules

A4

The biology of cell

Q5

What is anatomy?

Q6

What is physiology?

A5

The study of organization and structure of living organisms

A6

The study of functions and processes of living organisms

Q7

How are atoms, molecules, cells, tissues, organs, and organisms are related to each other?

Q8

List some of the organisms used in the biotechnology research.

A7

Atoms make up molecules such as carbohydrates, lipids, nucleic acids, and proteins.

Molecules are the building bocks of the smallest metabolically functional units of life called cells.

A group of cells make up a tissue, and tissues make up an organ.

Organs make up a living system called organism.

A8

- **Bacteria such as Escherichia coli (E. coli)**
- **Beans**
- **Cotton**
- **Cows**
- **Fruit flies**
- **Mice**
- **Worms**
- **Yeast**

Q9

What are organisms and microorganisms?

Q10

What is an organ?

A9

organism A living adaptive system of organs with organs interacting in such a way that they work as a single whole. You and tree are examples of organisms.

microorganism An organism that is too small to be seen by the human eye. Bacteria and fungi are examples of microorganisms.

A10

A collection of tissues that work together to perform a set of functions. Stomach and liver are examples.

Raw Materials of Biomanufacturing

Q11

What is a tissue?

Q12

What is a cell?

A11

A collection of interconnected cells functioning together within an organism with each cell performing a similar function. Muscle tissues and nervous tissue are examples.

A12

The smallest metabolically functional unit of life largely made of protein and DNA.

Q13

What is an adaptive system?

Q14

Describe the brief history of the premises of the cell theory.

A13

A system capable of learning from experience and changing accordingly.

A14

- **Mid 1600s.** An Englishman with the name of Robert Hooke observed tiny compartments in the cork that he examined through the newly invented microscope. He referred to these units as cells.

- **Late 1600s.** Anton Van Leeuwenhock, a Dutch merchant, studied cells in plants and animals.

- **1838.** Mathias Schleiden, a German botanist, proposed that all plants are composed of cells.

- **1839.** Theodore Schwann, a colleague of Mathias Schleiden, proposed that all animals like all plants, are also composed of cells.

- **1858.** Rudolf Virchow, a biologist, proposed that all living things are made of cells and that all cells form from already existing cells.

Q15

What are the two types of cells?

Q16

What is a cell composed of?

A15

Prokaryotic. These cells are usually singletons, that is, found in organisms composed of a single cell. An example is bacteria. These cells have no cell nucleus or membrane-bound compartments called organelles.

Eukaryotic. These cells are mostly found in multicellular organisms. A eukaryotic cell could be 1000 times larger in volume than a prokaryotic cell. These cells have cell nucleus and organelles.

A16

- **Nucleus.** Primarily composed of protein and DNA. DNA in a cell is organized into units called chromosomes.

- **Cytoplasm.** The complex of chemicals and structures exterior to the cell nuclus (in a eukaryotic cell). This is the space in which chemical reaction occur. Both eukaryotic and prokaryotic cells have cytoplasm.

- **Plasma membrane.** A bilayer of phsopholipis and proteins that surrounds the cytoplasm in a cell. Called cell membrane in case of a prokaryotic cell.

- **Cell wall.** A structure that contains carbohydrates and surrounds algal, fungal, and most procaryotic cells.

Q17

What are organelles?

Q18

List some examples of organelles.

A17

An organelle is a specialized compartment in the cytoplasm of a eukaryotic cell with a specific function.

A18

Centriole. Supports cell division.

Chloroplast. Supports the process of photosynthesis in green plants.

Cytoskeleton. Supports the cell shape and structure.

Endoplasmic reticulum (ER). Responsible for protein synthesis in the cell and transport of material from the cell.

Golgi body. Involved in the modification and sorting of proteins.

Lysosome. Contains enzymes to digest substances.

Mitochondria. Responsible for generating cellular energy.

Ribosome. Supports protein making.

Q19

What is an enzyme?

Q20

What are hormones?

A19

A kind of protein molecules that works as a catalyst in a chemical reaction, that is, helps bring about a chemical change without changing itself. Almost all reactions (processes) in a biological cell need enzymes to occur at significant speed.

A20

The messenger molecules that travel from cells to cells to regulate cellular functions. Hormones naturally exist in the body and are also one of the products of biotechnology companies.

Q21

What are chlorophylls?

Q22

What is photosynthesis?

A21

Green pigment molecules in plant cells used in photosynthesis. A pigment is a material that changes the color of light by reflecting some of its colors and absorbing others.

A22

A process by which plants and some bacteria use light energy to make organic food molecules such as carbohydrates from carbon dioxide and water

Q23

What is DNA?

Q24

What is a chromosome?

A23

Deoxyribonucleic acid, the genetic material that organisms inherit from their parents. A DNA molecule is a polymer made of monomers called nucleotides.

A24

A thread like linear strand that consists of a DNA molecule and the associated protein that serves to package and manage the DNA. In other words, a chromosome is a physically organized (or packaged) form of DNA.

Q25

What is a gene?

Q26

What are the four major molecule types in a cell?

A25

A section of DNA in a chromosome that makes a discrete unit of hereditary information

A26

- ♦ **Carbohydrates**
- ♦ **Lipids**
- ♦ **Nucleic acids**
- ♦ **Proteins**

Q27

What are carbohydrates?

Q28

What are the three kinds of carbohydrates?

A27

A carbohydrate is a compound molecule with carbon, hydrogen, and oxygen atoms in the ratio of 1:2:1, or a slight variation to it. Carbohydrates are the primary source of dietary energy for animals and are used as a building material in forming the plant body.

A28

- **Monosaccharides**
- **Disaccharides**
- **Polysaccharides**

Q29

What is a monosaccharide?

Q30

What is a disaccharide?

A29

A simple carbohydrate molecule that cannot be broken further into smaller carbohydrate molecules. Monosaccharide molecules are used as monomers to form polymers of more complex carbohydrates.

Examples:

- **Glucose.** Sugar produced during photosynthesis.

- **Fructose.** The sugar that gives honey its sweet taste.

A30

A disaccharide is a molecule formed from binding two monosaccharide molecules through dehydration reaction, that is, by losing a water molecule.

Examples:

Lactose. A sugar that gives milk its slightly sweet taste.

Sucrose. Cane sugar.

Raw Materials of Biomanufacturing

Q31

What is a polysaccharide?

Q32

What are lipids?

A31

A polysaccharide is a complex carbohydrate, a polymer made of monosaccharide monomers. Because of their long polymer structure, polysaccharides are suitable to work as structural and energy storage molecules.

Examples:

♦ **Starch.** Used by plants to store large amounts of glucose.

♦ **Cellulose.** Structural carbohydrate; provides structural support in plant cell walls. Wood, paper, and cotton are largely cellulose.

A32

A lipid is an organic compound largely composed of carbon and hydrogen atoms and thereby is also called a hydrocarbon. They are insoluble in water, that is, *hydrophobic*. Fats, plant oils, and cholesterol are some examples.

Q33

What are phospholipids?

Q34

What is a nucleic acid?

A33

A type of lipids found in the cell walls

A34

A polymer composed of nucleotides as monomers. This chain of nucleotides conveys the genetic information. There are two types of nucleic acids:

- ♦ **Deoxyribonucleic acid (DNA).**

- ♦ **Ribonucleic acid (RNA).**

Q35

What is a nucleotide?

Q36

What is a nitrogenous base?

A35

A component (monomer) of a nucleic acid composed of a carbohydrate molecule, a phosphate group, and a nitrogenous base.

A36

Nitrogen-containing compounds found in nucleotides.

Q37

What are proteins?

Q38

What is a polypeptide?

A37

A protein is a polymer composed of amino acids as monomers. The bond between adjacent amino acids is called a peptide bond. The chain itself is called a polypeptide and usually consists of 100 or more amino acid molecules. Each amino acid in a protein comes from a group of 20 amino acids called alpha amino acids.

A38

Any polymer composed of any amino acids as monomers. A protein is a polypeptide whose monomers are alpha amino acids.

Q39

What are proteins good for?

Q40

What is the gel-like liquid composed of thousands of molecules suspended in water outside the nucleus of a cell?

A39

Contractile proteins. Found in muscles.

Storage proteins. Source of amino acids to develop plants and animals. Found in eggs and seeds.

Structural proteins. Provide support. Examples: Proteins found in feathers, hair, horns, and spider webs.

Transport proteins. An example is hemoglobin in blood that takes oxygen from your lungs to other parts of the body.

A40

Cytoplasm

Q41

What is the 6-carbon carbohydrate that is produced by plants during photosynthesis and is used as a source of energy by animals including human?

Q42

These are the molecules that are colored due to the light of specific wavelength that they reflect:

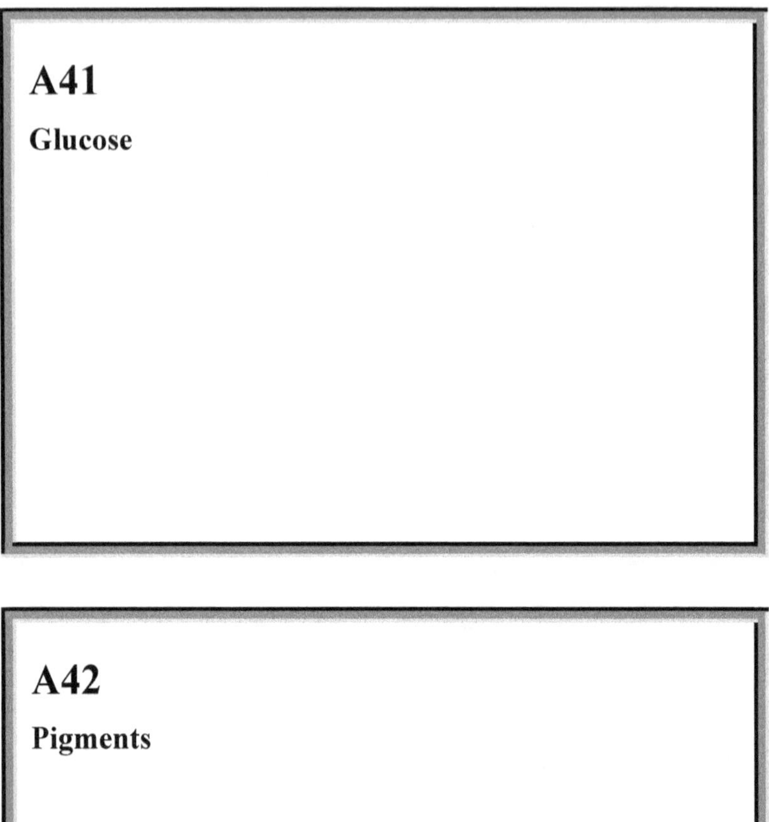

A41

Glucose

A42

Pigments

Q1

What is a solution?

Q2

You dissolved some sodium chloride (table salt) in water. Identify solution, solute, and solvent in this mixture.

A1

A homogeneous mixture of two or more substances prepared by dissolving one substance into another. The relevant terms are:

- **Solute.** The substance that is dissolved

- **Solvent.** The substance in which the solute is dissolved.

A2

Solution. The mixture itself

Solute. Sodium chloride

Solvent. Water

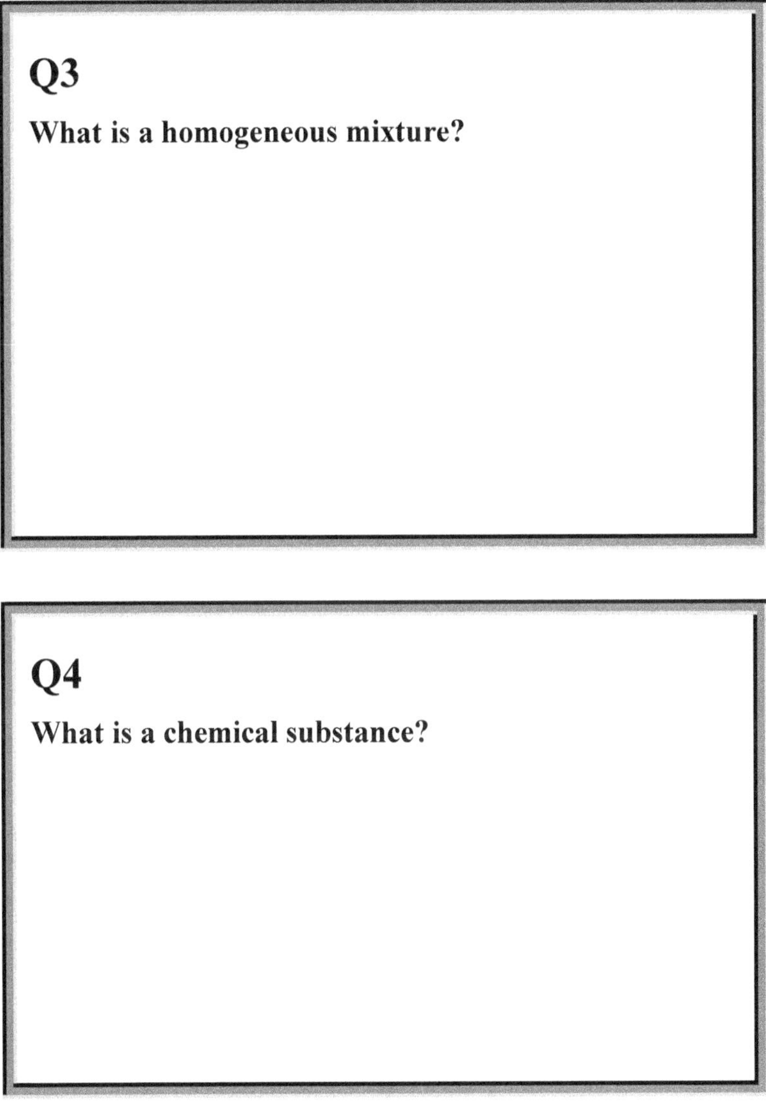

Q3
What is a homogeneous mixture?
Q4
What is a chemical substance?

A3

A mixture of two or more pure chemical substances that has a uniform appearance and uniform properties throughout

A4

A (pure) chemical substance (also called pure substance or just a substance) is a material with a definite chemical composition, that is, all samples of the substance have the same composition. A pure substance cannot be separated into other substances without a chemical reaction. Pure water is an example of a chemical substance.

Q5

Solutes are not always solid. Assume you dilute 90% methyl alcohol (methanol) to 70% by adding some water to it. Identify the solute and the solvent in this solution.

Q6

What is the proportion of solute and solvent in a 10% solution?

A5

Solute. Methanol

Solvent. Water

A6

Solution. 100 parts
Solute. 10 parts
Solvent. 90 parts

Q7

Can you make a solution of lipids by using water as a solvent?

Q8

What is concentration of a solution?

A7

Most of the lipids are not soluble in water. You will need a solvent in which lipids are soluble such as ethanol or acetone.

A8

The ratio of the mass of the solute in a given volume of the solution:
Concentratio = Mass of the solute/Volume of the solution

You need to be careful and consistent about the units of mass and vlume.

Q9

Name the different ways to measure concentration of a solution.

Q10

What are the common units of concentration in the method of density?

A9

- **Density, that is, mass/volume**
- **Percent density**
- **Molarity**
- **Normality**

A10

- g/L
- mg/mL
- µg/mL
- µg/µL

Q11

You disolved 16.8 g of salt in water to make 2 L of sodium chloride solution. What is the concentration of this solution?

Q12

What is molecular weight of a substance?

A11

Concentration = 16.8 g/2L = 8.4 g/L
You can also write it as:
  Concentration = 8.4 mg/mL
                = 8.4 μg/μL

A12

The mass of one molecule of the substance. It's also
called molecular mass, and is usually measured in atomic
mass units (amu).

Q13

What is an atomic mass unit?

Q14

What is a mole?

A13

One twelfth of the mass of an unbound atom of carbon (C-12) at rest. An atom of hydrogen weighs 1.01 (about 1) amu. The atomic mass units of elements are shown in the periodic table with their symbols.

A14

A mole of any substance is the amount of the substance that contains the number of molecules of the substance equal to the Avogadro's number, which is about 6.022×10^{23}.

Q15

What is the molecular weight of sodium chloride (NaCl)?

Q16

What is the realtionship between a mole and the molecular weight?

A15

Molecular weight of Na = 22.99 amu
Molecular weight of Cl = 35.45 amu
Molecular weight of NaCl = 22.99 amu+ 35.45 amu =
58.44 amu

A16

The weight of a mole of a substabce is equal to the
molecular weight of the same substance; amu
replaced with g.

Q17

What is the weight of one mole of NaCl?

Q18

What is the molecular weight of NaCl in units of grams?

A17

58.44 g because the molecular weight of NaCl is 58.44 amu.

A18

Molecular weight = Weight of one molecule
= Weight of one mole /
      Number of molecules in the mole
= 58.44 g / $(6.022 \times 10^{23}$ molecules)
= 9.70×10^{-23} g/molecule

Q19

You disolved 16.88 g of salt in water to make 2 L of sodium chloride solution. What is the concentration of this solution measured in molarity?

Q20

How will you prepare a 2L volume of 0.1444 M NaCl solution?

A19

Concentration = 16.88 g/2L
  = (16.88 g/2L) x (mole/58.44 g)
  = 0.1444 mole/L
  = 0.1444 M

A20

1. Weigh 16.88 g (0.2888 moles) of NaCl.
2. Place NaCl in a suitable container.
3. Add some water in it.
4. Stir to dissolve.
5. Keep adding water and dissolving until the volume becomes 2L.

Q21

You want to dilute a concentrated solution. Which equation will be helpful?

Q22

How will you make 2.00L litre of 10.0g/L NaCl solution from 20.0 g/L concentrated soltion?

A21

$C_c V_c = C_d V_d$

Where C_c and V_c are the concentration and volume of the concentrated solution, and C_d and V_d are the concentration and volume for the diluted solution. This equation holds because the amount of the solute in the concentrated solution and the diluted solution is the same.

A22

$C_c V_c = C_d V_d$

$\Rightarrow$

$$V_c = C_d V_d / C_c$$
$$= (10.0 \text{g/L}) * (2.00 \text{L}) / (20.0 \text{ g/L})$$
$$= 1.00 \text{ L}$$

This means:
1. Take 1.00 L of the concentrated solution.
2. Add enough water to it to make it 2 L.

Q23

What is buffer?

Q24

What is pH?

A23

A buffer solution is a solution that resists a change in pH.

A24

A measure of the acidity of a solution. It's calculated as a funtion of H^+ ions in the solution.

Q25

What are some of the tools to measure volumes in a biotechnology lab?

Q26

How precisely can you measure mass in a biotechnology lab?

A25

- **Graduated cylinder.** 10 mL to 2L

- **Pipet.** 0.1 mL to 50 mL

- **Micropipet.** 0.5 μL to 1 mL

A26

Most analytical balances with electronic display can measure mass down to milligrams.

Q27

You add 40.0 mL of water to 20.0 mL of 0.750 M NaOH. What is the concentration in molarity of the diluted solution?

Q28

You want to prepare 5.00 L 0.500 M HCL. How much of commercially available 11.0 M Hcl will you need?

A27

$M_1 V_1 = M_2 V_2$

$\Rightarrow$

$M_2 = M_1 V_1 / V_2$
   $= 0.750 \text{ M} \times 20.0 \text{ mL} / 60.0 \text{ mL}$
   $= 0.250 \text{ M}$

A28

$M_1 V_1 = M_2 V_2$

$\Rightarrow$

$V_1 = M_2 V_2 / M_1$
   $= 0.500 \text{M} \times 5.00 \text{ L} / 11.0 \text{M}$
   $= 0.227 \text{ L}$

This means:

1. Take 0.227 L of the concentrated (11.0M) solution.
2. Add enough water to it to make it 5.00 L.

Q1

What is genetics?

Q2

What is gene expression?

A1

The science of heredity and hereditary variations. In other words, it's a study of genes and how they are inherited and expressed.

A2

Gene expression is the process in which an RNA and then a protein is synthesized according to the information coded in the gene.

Q3

Which two DNA related techniques triggered the current biotechnology revolution?

Q4

The abilities to transfer genes between cells and thereby trick cells to create specific proteins have made possible what kinds of products?

A3

- **Transfer DNA between cells**

- **Trick (manipulate) the cells to create specific proteins by introducing the corresponding DNA into them**

A4

- **Cellular proteins**

- **Tissues**

- **Organs**

- **Organisms with new or modified characteristics**

Q5

What is the role of proteins in a cell?

Q6

What determines how will a protein be synthesized?

A5

Proteins are the work horses of the cells and they give cells and the organisms their unique characteristics.

A6

The genetic code in the DNA

 Introduction to Genetics

Q7

What in a DNA molecule determines the genetic information?

Q8

What is the central dogma of molecular biology?

A7

The sequence of nucleotides

A8

The central dogma of molecular biology describes how the genetic information is used in synthesizing proteins:

1. **DNA Replication.** DNA is copied to DNA for inheritance.

2. **Transcription.** The information contained in a part of DNA is transferred to newly created messenger RNA (mRNA).

3. **Translation.** The mRNA moves into ribosome where it is translated to synthesize protein.

          Introduction to Genetics

Q9

What is the genome of an organism?

Q10

How does genome vary within a species?

A9

The entire sum of DNA in the cell including genes and non-coding sequences.

A10

It varies from organism to organism. However, all the cells except the sex cells within an organism carry the same genome. Yet, all cells in the same organism are not the same, as they have acquired specific functionalities through a process called cell differentiation.

Q11

What is the basis of DNA fingerprinting?

Q12

DNA and RNA are two types of nucleic acids. What is a nucleic acid?

A11

The genomic loci and the length of certain types of small repetitive sequences vary significantly from human to human.

A12

A nucleic acid is a polymer composed from monomers called nucleotides.

Q13

What is a nucleotide?

Q14

Each nucleotide in DNA has the same sugar and phosphate group. So, the four kinds of nucleotides are distinguished by the four different nitrogenous bases. Each nucleotide contains one these four nitrogenous bases. What are these four kinds of nitrogenous bases?

A13

A nucleotide is a compound molecule with the following structure:

♦ **A five-carbon sugar at the center: deoxyribose in DNA and ribose in RNA**

♦ **Negatively charged phosphate group attached to the sugar**

♦ **A base containing nitrogen, nitrogenous base, attached to the sugar**

Each DNA molecule is composed of two strands, and each strand is a polynucleotide composed of four different kinds of nucleotides.

A14

♦ **Adenine (A).** A double ring structure of carbon, hydrogen, and nitrogen atoms: $C_5H_5N_5$

♦ **Guanine (G).** A double ring structure of carbon, hydrogen, and nitrogen atoms: $C_5H_5N_5O$

♦ **Cytosine (C).** A single ring structure of carbon, hydrogen, nitrogen, and oxygen atoms: $C_4H_5N_3O$

♦ **Thymine (T).** A single ring structure of carbon, hydrogen, nitrogen, and oxygen atoms: $C_5H_6N_2O_2$

     Introduction to Genetics

Q15

What keeps the two strands of a DNA molecule together?

Q16

What are some of the variations among DNA molecules from different organisms?

A15

The hydrogen bonds (H-bonds) between the nitrogenous bases of the two strands. Only two base pairings are possible:

- A-T

- C-G

A16

- The length of a DNA strand, say, in base pair (bp) units.

- The number of DNA strands in a cell, that is, the number of chromosomes

- The sequence of different kinds of nucleotides in the DNA strand that makes the genetic code

- The package shape of a DNA strand, e.g., circular or linear

Q17

Where in the body of an organism is the DNA made?

Q18

What is a cell culture?

A17

DNA is made in cells. Biotechnologists can get cells from nature or they can create a cell culture in the lab.

A18

The environment and process used to grow cells under controlled conditions

 Introduction to Genetics

Q19

Where does DNA reside in a prokaryotic cell?

Q20

What is a plasmid?

A19

Floating in the cytoplasm

A20

A ring shaped DNA (separate from the chromosomal DNA) found in prokaryotes and yeasts

 Introduction to Genetics

Q21

What are vectors?

Q22

What are R plasmids?

Introduction to Genetics

Q23

What is an operon?

Q24

How does an operon work to produce an mRNA?

A23

A unit of DNA, common in prokaryotes, that contains operator, promoter and structural genes with related functions, which are controlled as a unit to produce messenger RNA (mRNA)

A24

1. **Process starts in the region at the beginning of a structural gene.**

2. **RNA polymerase, an enzyme to synthesize the mRNA molecule, attaches to DNA at the promoter.**

3. **This turns on the gene.**

4. **The RNA polymerase makes its way down the DNA strand to the (structural) gene.**

5. **At the structural gene, the RNA polymerase develops an mRNA from the free floating nucleotides. This mRNA is decoded to build a peptide at a ribosome.**

     Introduction to Genetics

Q25

What enables the bacteria cells to make only certain proteins at certain times?

Q26

What is agar?

A25

**By blocking and unblocking the RNA polymerase
from traveling down the DNA strand to the structural
gene.** Blocking is facilitated by a region called operator
that is located just before the structural gene:

1. A regulatory molecule attaches to the operator.

2. The operon is turned off.

3. The RNA polymerase is stopped from traveling down
    to the structural gene.

A26

**A solid substance used as a solid culture medium to
grow bacteria and fungi**

Introduction to Genetics

Q27

What is sterilization?

Q28

What is the sterile technique?

A27

A process to eliminate the unwanted agents such as bacteria or fungi from a specific area such as equipment, food, biological culture medium, or a surface. Sterilization can be achieved through applications of chemicals, filtration, or heat.

A28

A process of doing something without contamination by an unwanted organism, cell, or the like

Q29

What is a growth medium?

Q30

What is media preparation?

A29

A substance in which cells or microorganisms can grow. Different kinds of media can be used to grow different kinds of cells. Media are used to develop cultures such as a cell culture. So, a growth medium is also called culture medium.

A30

The process of preparing a specific growth medium by combining and sterilizing the ingredients.

Q31

What is an agar plate?

Q32

How is eukaryotic DNA similar to prokaryotic DNA?

A31

A sterile dish, called Petri dish, that contains nutrients in addition to agar and is used to create bacteria or fungi culture. It's a shallow cylindrical dish made of glass or plastic.

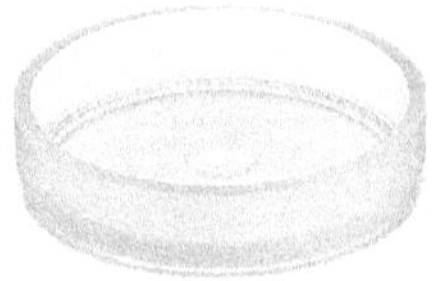

Image: courtesy of www.sciencegear.com

A32

♦ **Same double helix structures with two strands made of repeating nucleotides and bound to each other by H-bonds**

♦ **Uses the same basis for code: A, C, G, and T.**

Q33

How is eukaryotic DNA different from prokaryotic DNA?

Q34

How does the number of chromosomes vary within a species and among different species?

A33

- DNA in a eukaryotic cell is packaged into thread like structures called chromosomes. A chromosome in a prokaryotic cell is usually of circular shape.

- The genome of eukaryotes is substantially larger than that of prokaryotes.

A34

- Each cell in an organism carries the same number of chromosomes.

- Number of chromosomes in a cell varies from species to species.

For example, humans have 46 chromosomes per cell, and a common fruit fly has only 8.

Q35

What is the spacer DNA?

Q36

What is an exon?

A35

The non-coding DNA material that fills the space in between genes in the DNA sequence. Majority of the DNA in human genome is the spacer DNA.

A36

A coding portion of a gene, that is, the portion that is expressed

   Introduction to Genetics

Q37

What is an intron?

Q38

What is a histone?

A37

A portion of a gene that is transcribed into an mRNA molecule, but is not expressed. Introns sit between exons in a gene, whereas spacer DNA sits between genes.

A38

A protein molecule that plays a role in DNA packing in a eukaryotic chromosome.

Q39

What is a virus?

Q40

How are viruses used in biotechnology?

A39

A nano (or sub-microscopic) particle that has the capability of infecting cells of living organisms. A virus contains genetic material protected in a protein coat. Viruses usually range from 20 to 300 nm in size. Unlike cells, viruses cannot multiply on their own, and can only replicate themselves by infecting a host cell.

A40

- **Because viruses infect the living organisms, they are often the target of the biotechnology solutions such as products and therapies.**

- **Virus particles are used in biotechnology research to carry DNA from one cell to another.**

Q41

What is gene therapy?

Q42

What is genetic engineering?

A41

The treatment of a disease by providing the patient with a new gene, for example, replacing dysfunctional genes with functional genes. It's also called human gene therapy.

A42

The scientific way of altering genes or genetic materials for the purpose of either creating new desirable traits in organisms or to eliminate the undesirable traits

Introduction to Genetics

Q43

What is the general process of genetic engineering?

Q44

What is recombinant DNA?

A43

1. Identify the molecules that need to be produced through genetic engineering.

2. Isolate the DNA (gene) that contains the instructions to produce the identified molecules.

3. Manipulate the DNA instructions to produce the desirable product. This can be accomplished by one of the following two ways:

   - Change the DNA instructions inside the cells of the target organism.

   - Introduce the new instructions into the cells of another organism that can produce the desired molecules more efficiently.

4. Manufacture the molecules (product).

5. Test the molecules for their new traits.

A44

A DNA molecule carrying genes from two or more sources combined through genetic engineering.

Introduction to Genetics

Q1

What is a protein?

Q2

What is the role of proteins in biotechnology?

A1

A polymer molecule, an important component of a cell, composed of amino acids as monomers.

A2

Protein molecules are either products themselves or are important components of most of the products in the biotechnology industry.

Q3

List some tools and techniques that the researchers use to study the functions and structures of proteins.

Q4

What is the basic structure of a protein molecule?

A3

Mass spectrometer. Used to measure the molecular mass of a protein molecule.

X-ray crystallography. Used to explore the three dimensional structure of a protein molecule.

Behavior analysis. Used to determine the physical and chemical properties of a protein molecule such as electric charge and solubility.

A4

♦ **A protein molecule is a polymer composed of amino acids as monomers.**

♦ **The amino acids in a protein molecules are bonded together through bonds called peptide bonds.**

Q5

What is a peptide bond?

Q6

What is a polypeptide chain?

A5

The bond between the carboxyl group of one amino acid and the amino group of the other amino acid.

A6

The chain formed by peptide bonds in a protein molecule

Proteins in Biotechnology

Q7

What is an amino acid?

Q8

What distinguishes one amino acid from another?

A7

A molecule with a carbon atom at the center connected to a carboxyl group (COOH) on one side and an amino group (NH_2) on the other side. An amino acid also has a group called an R-group.

A8

The R-group, which may have properties such as charged or uncharged, water soluble or not, and polar or nonpolar

   Proteins in Biotechnology

Q9

Give some examples of amino acids along with their R-groups.

Q10

How many amino acids a protein may have?

A9

Amino Acid	Properties	R-group
Alanine $C_3H_7NO_2$	nonpolar, neutral	CH_3
Arginine $C_6H_{14}N_4O_2$	polar, positively charged	$HN=C(NH_2)-NH$
Glycine $C_3H_5NO_2$	nonpolar, neutral	H
Aspartic acid $C_4H_7NO_4$	polar, negatively charged	$HOOC-CH_2$

A10

Large number: could be up to hundereds

Proteins in Biotechnology

Q11

How many amino acids in total there are that can participate in composing the chain in a protein?

Q12

Name some protein types (groups) by functions.

A11

Twenty amino acids called aplha amino acids

A12

Protein type	Examples
antibody	**HER2 antibody**. Recognizes a breast cancer protein. **Gamma globulin**. Recognizes a whole variety of foreign proteins.
enzyme	**amylase**. Converts starch to sugar. **alcohol dehydrogenase**. Breaks down alcohol which could otherwise be toxic.
hormone	**insulin**. Regulates blood sugar. Also used to treat some forms of diabetes.
structural	**collagen.** Component of bones and skin.
transport	**hemoglobin**. Carries oxygen in the blood stream.

 Proteins in Biotechnology

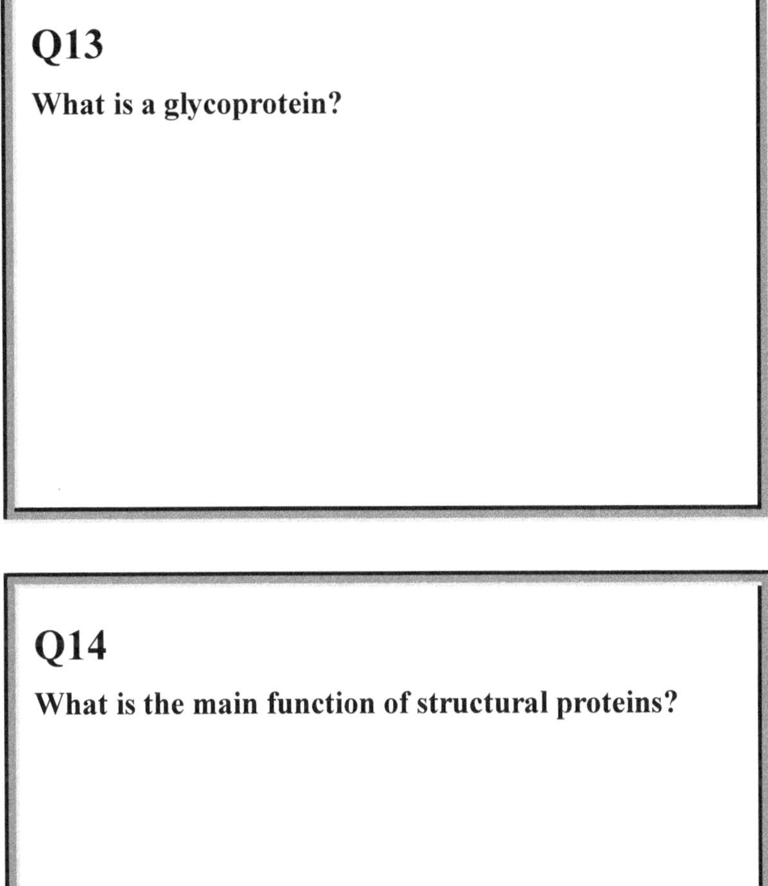

Q13

What is a glycoprotein?

Q14

What is the main function of structural proteins?

A13

A molecule made of a protein and a carbohydrate. In other words, it's a protein which has sugar groups added to it.

A14

To provide support (or stiffness). Examples are the proteins in bones, feathers, hair, connective tissues, horns, and spider webs.

Q15

What is the main function of antibody proteins?

Q16

What is an immune system?

A15

To recognize and bind molecules of foreign substances in the body and traget them for destruction. Antibodies are part of the adaptive immune system.

A16

The system of cells in a body that protetcts the body by recognizing and attacking specific types of pathogens (disease-causing cells) and cancer cells

Q17

What is epitope?

Q18

What is ELISA?

A17

The specific region of a molecule to which an antibody binds

A18

Enzyme-linked immunospecific assay. A technique used to measure the amount of protein (or antibody) in a solution.

Q19

What are monoclonal antibodies?

Q20

What are hybridoma cells?

A19

Monoclonal antibodies are the identical antibodies produced by one type of immune cell and are all clones of the single parent cell.

It is possible to produce monoclonal antibodies for a given substance to bind to that substance. These antibodies can be used to detect or purify the given substance.

A20

The cells engineered to produce monoclonal antibodies in large amounts

Q21

Where in the human body is protein produced?

Q22

What is protein synthesis?

A21

Protein synthesis occurs inside a cell. During its lifetime, a typical cell produces millions of protein molecules which fall into more than 2000 different categories.

A22

The creation of proteins from the amino acids by using DNA and RNA. In a cell, the protein synthesis occurs through transcription and translation.

 Proteins in Biotechnology

Q23

What is transcription?

Q24

What is the translation during protein synthesis?

A23

The process of transferring genetic information from DNA to RNA, which is produced during the process. Messenger RNA (mRNA) is a product of transcription.

A24

The process of syntesizing polypeptides from amino acids by using the genetic information encoded in an mRNA molecule

Q25

List the basic steps in the process of protein synthesis in a cell.

Q26

What are the two main uses of enzymes in biotechnology?

A25

1. The structural genes in a DNA molecule of a
    chromosome carries the instructions to generate
    protein.

2. During gene expression, a structural gene is
    rewritten as messenger RNA (mRNA), a process
    called transcription.

3. The mRNA floats to a ribosome.

4. At the ribosome, the mRNA code is tranlated to
    compile a polypeptide chain of amino acids.

5. Due to attractive and repulsive forces caused by
    the R-groups in amino acids, the polypeptide
    chain is spontaneously folded into a protein.

A26

1. Catalyze chemical reactions

2. Control steps in the breakdown and production of
    biotech products

Proteins in Biotechnology

Q27

The molecules on which enzymes act are called what?

Q28

List some examples of enzyme types.

A27

Substrates

A28

Enzyme Group	Examples	General Funtcion
hydrolases	Dnase, lactase, sucrase	catalyze hydrolysis reactions, that is, break down of polymer molcules into smaller molecules by adding water
isomerases	fructose isomerase	Catalyze reactions that involve interconversion of polymers such as: $A \rightarrow B$
lyases	pectase	Split the substrates
synthetases	ATP synthetase, DNA polymerases, RNA polymerases	Combine smaller molecules into larger ones
transferases	hexokinase	Catalyze transfer of an organic group from one compound to another

  Proteins in Biotechnology

Q29

What is a cofactor?

Q30

What is a coenzyme?

A29

A non-protein substance such as an ion or a coenzyme that is required to be associated with an enzyme in order for the enzyme to function

A30

An organic molecule, usually a vitamin or a compund synthesized from a vitamin, that acts as a cofactor to support an enzyme to catalyze a reaction

Q31

What factors affect an enzyme's activity and effectiveness?

Q32

List the values of pH on the scale of 0 to 14 for some common substances.

A31

- **Concentration.** Amount of substance in a solution affects how quickly enzymes work
- **Temprature.** Each enzyme has an optimum temperature at which its activitiy is maximum.
- **pH. Potential hydrogen.** Each enzyme has an optimum value of pH at which it works the best. The pH is the degree of acidity of a solution. The pH scale goes from 0 (for highest acidity) to 14 (for lowest acidity). In other words, pH is a measure of H^+ ions concentration in a solution.

A32

Substance	pH
Lemon juice	2.4
Tomato juice	4
Pure water	7
Human blood	7.4
Solution inside most living cells	7
Household bleach	Between 12 and 13

Solutions with pH equal to 7 are neutral, less than 7 are acids, and greater than 7 are bases.

Proteins in Biotechnology

Q33

What is an acid?

Q34

What is a base?

A33

A chemical compound that releases H$^+$ ion to a solution

A34

A compound that accepts (or removes) H$^+$ ions from a solution

Q35

What properties of proteins are exploited by the researchers to separate them from other molecules?

Q36

What is PAGE?

A35

- ◆ **Amino acid composition**
- ◆ **Net charge**
- ◆ **Size and shape**
- ◆ **Solubility**

A36

Polyacrylamide gel electrophoresis. A technique used to separate molecules such as protein, DNA, and RNA by using electric charge.

Q37

What is the protein profiling of a cell?

Q38

How does protein profile help identify a disease?

A37

Identification and quantification of all the proteins in the cell

A38

Comparing the profiles of a cell with another may explain the observed differences in the functions and structures of the cells, and thereby help the researchers understand a dissease related to the structure or function of a cell type.

Q39

How can protein manipulation techniques be used to remove certain tumors?

Q40

What is the main cause of most of the genetic disorders?

A39

Starving the tumors of their blood supply by blocking certain kind of proteins

A40

Certain activities or a lack of certain activities of various proteins

Q41

How do proteins help in determinig the evolutionary history of species?

Q42

Human with THIS disease has abnormally shaped red blood cells:

A41

Proteins are syntesized according to the instructions in the DNA. Therefore, the degree of similarities (or differences) in proteins indicates the similarities (or differences) in the DNA, which carries hereditary information.

A42

Sickle cell disease

Proteins in Biotechnology

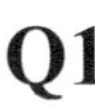

Q1

List some areas of biotechnology products.

Q2

List some sources of biotechnology products.

A1

- **Agricultural products**
- **Industrial products**
- **Pharmaceutical products**
- **Research related products such as tools and data**

A2

- **Organisms**
- **Organs**
- **Cells**
- **Molecules such as proteins and DNA**

Q3

What is t-PA?

Q4

What is a Chinese Hamster?

A3

Tissue plasminogen activator; An enzyme that clears blocked blood vessels by breaking down blood clots; one of the first genetically engineered products

A4

A species of hamsters

   Biotechnology Products

Q5

What is a CHO cell?

Q6

What is an ovary?

A5

Chinese Hamster ovary cell; a cell line derived from the Chinese Hamster ovary cells; often used in biological and medical research

A6

A reproductive organ of female organisms that produces eggs

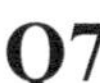

Q7

True or false: Biotechnologists cloned the human t-PA gene in CHO cells.

Q8

What are antibiotics?

A7

True

A8

Molecular agents naturally produced by a few bacterial and fungal species that inhibits or kills other microorganisms

Q9

List some diseases cured by antibiotics.

Q10

True or false: With advances in organic chemistry and biotechnology, many antibiotics can now be produced through chemical synthesis.

A9

- **Bronchitis**
- **Pneumonia**
- **Strep throat**

A10

True

Q11

True or false: Some biotechnology products are derived directly from living organisms in nature; some are cloned in genetically engineered organisms; while others are made through chemical synthesis.

Q12

The molecules of THIS enzyme break starch into sugar, and this was one of the first biotechnology products on the market:

A11

True

A12

Amylase

Q13

True or false: Many microorganisms produce amylase. For this reason, biotechnologists are interested in using Bacillus subtilis and E. coli as hosts to produce amylase.

Q14

What is an assay?

A13

True

A14

A procedure (or test) used to examine or analyze a substance for characteristics such as existence, concentration, composition, or quality

Q15

A procedure (or experiment) designed to demonstrate that an enzyme is conducting the expected reaction is called an:

Q16

An experiment designed to determine the number of moles of a solute in a solution is called a:

A15

Activity assay

A16

Concentration assay

Q17

What is ELISA?

Q18

The problem with using antibiotics is that some bacteria develop resistance to the action of many antibiotics; these bacteria are then considered:

A17

Enzyme Linked Immuno Sorbent Assay; a technique used to detect the presence of an antibody (or antigen) in a sample

A18

Antibiotic resistant

Q19

What is an antimicrobial?

Q20

What is antiseptic?

A19

A substance that either kills or inhibits the growth of one or more microorganisms such as bacteria, fungi, or viruses

A20

An antimicrobial substance, such as alcohol or iodine, that is used to clean surfaces including the surface of a human body by reducing or killing microorganisms

Q21

Distinguish between antibiotics, antiseptic, and disinfectants.

Q22

How does recombinant DNA work for producing protein?

A21

Antibiotics destroy microorganisms within a body, antiseptics destroy microorganisms on a living tissue (surface), whereas disinfectants destroy microorganisms on non-living objects.

A22

1. **The DNA containing the genes for the production of the desired protein is added to a cell line in the laboratory.**

2. **The cells start reading the DNA and produce the protein accordingly.**

Biotechnology Products

Q23

The manufacturing guidelines from food and drug administration (FDA) to ensure safety and purity are called:

Q24

A set of instructions to describe a procedure or sets of procedures to perform an operation is called:

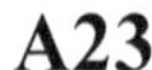

A23

GMP; good manufacturing practices.

A24

Standard Operating Procedure; SOP.

Q25

Giving the final shape to a product such as powder or tablet is called:

Q26

A genetically engineered cell such as a cell to which a foreign material has been introduced:

A25

Formulation

A26

Transfection

Q27

What is pathogenesis?

Q28

What is medicine?

A27

The mechanism through which a disease is caused and developed; pathos means disease and genesis means development.

A28

Anything used in treating a disease or illness to restore health

Q29

What is a drug?

Q30

What is drug discovery?

A29

Broader definition: A substance that alters normal bodily function.

Pharmacological definition: A chemical substance used in the prevention, diagnosis, cure, or treatment of diseases, or used just to enhance physical or mental wellness.

A30

The process of identifying drugs (molecules) that will treat a disease

Q31

What is drug delivery?

Q32

What is organic synthesis?

A31

The delivery of a pharmaceutical compoud (drug) inside a living body such as that of human

A32

The process of synthesising drug molecules in a laboratory from simpler molecules

Q33

The chemistry that deals with the rapid synthesis of larger organic molecules from the smaller ones:

Q34

What is parallel synthesis?

A33

Combinatorial chemistry

A34

A process of producing a large number of batches of same or similar compounds (such as drugs) simultaneously

Q35

What is a library in biotechnology?

Q36

What is a microarray?

A35

A well managed collection of compounds such as DNA molecules and proteins

A36

A system that consists of small components arrayed on a solid surface

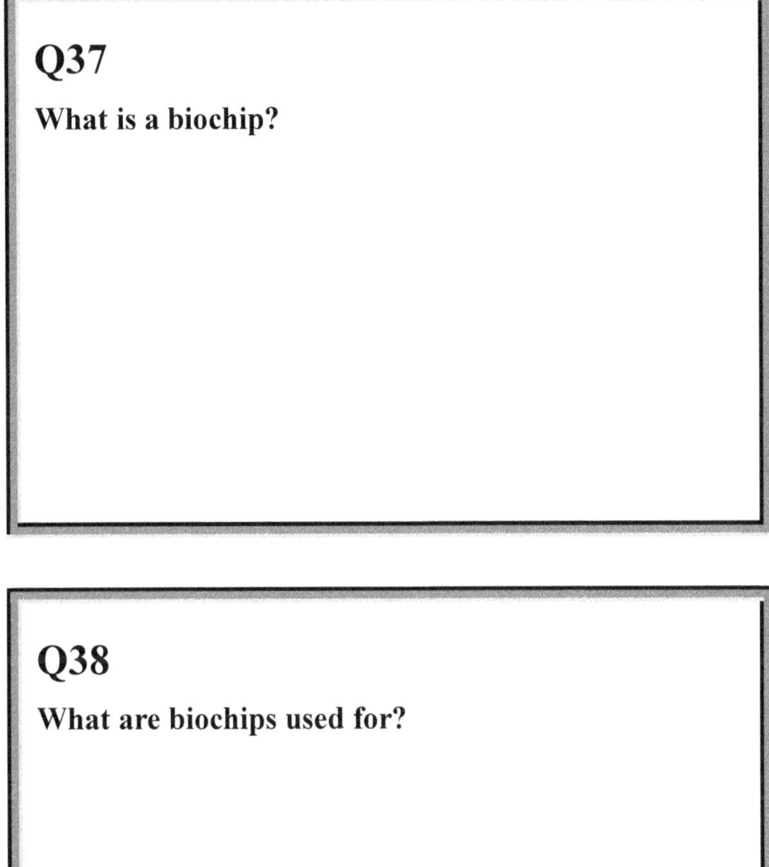

Q37

What is a biochip?

Q38

What are biochips used for?

A37

A microarray in which the components are bio particles such as DNA molecules or proteins. In other words, it's an integrated circuit composed of biochemical molecules.

A38

To produce patient profile by performing a panel of related tests on a single sample

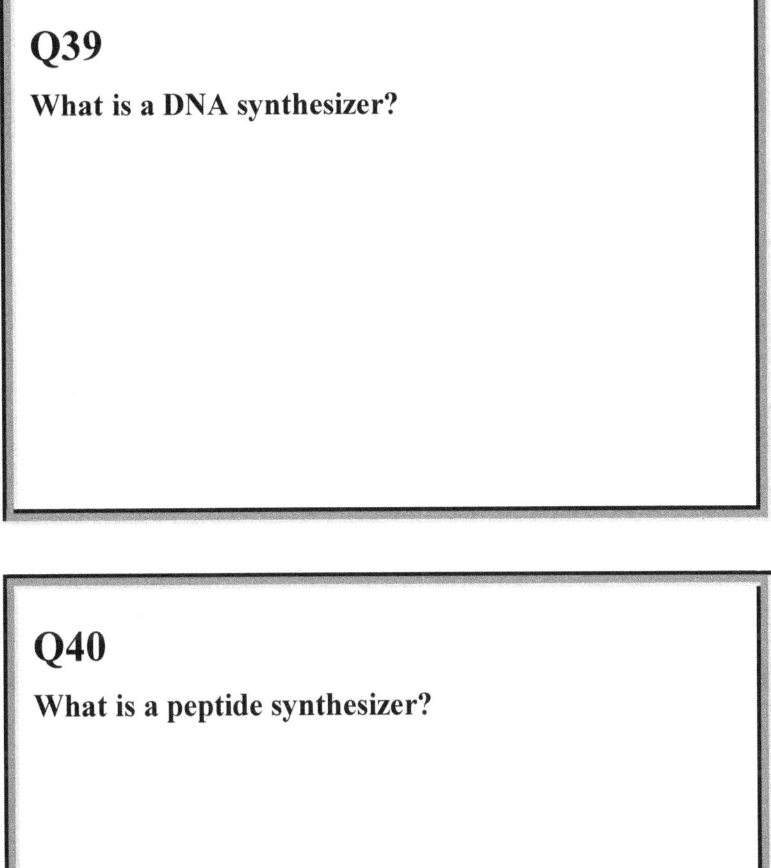

Q39

What is a DNA synthesizer?

Q40

What is a peptide synthesizer?

A39

An instrument used to produce short segments of DNA

A40

An instrument used to produce peptides; chains of amino acids that compose proteins.

Q41

What is a vaccine?

Q42

What is a pathogen?

A41

A harmless derivative or variant of a pathogen used to stimulate a host organism's immune system to build a long term defense against a specific pathogen.

A42

An organism that causes a disease

Q1

List some of the tools and techniques of biotechnology.

Q2

True or false: Most microbial agents are in the size range of micrometers, and therefore light (optical) microscopes are used to observe them.

A1

- **Light microscope**
- **Staining**
- **Spectrometers**
- **Recombinant DNA**
- **DNA sequencing**
- **Chromatography**
- **PCR**
- **Sterilization**
- **Electrophoresis**

A2

True

Q3

What is the formula for the resolving power, P_R, of a microscope?

Q4

The numerical aperture of the objective lens of your light microscope is 1.25. The average wavelength of white light is about 500 nm. What is the minimum size of a particle that you can see with this microscope as a clear and distinct particle?

A3

$$P_R = \frac{\lambda}{2N_A}$$

where λ is the wavelength of light used in the microscope, and N_A is the numerical aperture of the microscope's objective lens.

A4

$$P_R = \frac{\lambda}{2\,N_A}$$

$$= \frac{500nm}{2*1.25}$$

$$= 200nm$$

$$= 0.200\,\mu m$$

So, the average resolving power of this light microscope is 0.200 μm. Therefore, on average, the smallest size of a particle that can be clearly and distinctively seen with this microscope is 0.200 μm.

Note: 1 μm = 1000 nm

Tools and Techniques of Biotechnology

Q5

The cytoplasm of bacterial cells lack color and therefore makes it hard to view the cells against a bright background in a light microscope. For this reason, biotechnologists stain bacterial cells with a dye before viewing them. These techniques are called:

Q6

These staining techniques allow to differentiate bacterial cells into two groups based on the staining differences between them:

A5

Staining techniques

A6

Differential staining techniques

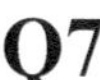

Q7

This differential staining technique is used to identify bacterial cells as gram negative or gram positive:

Q8

What is gram negative?

A7

Gram stain

A8

A bacterial cell that stains red (or pink) after Gram staining

 Tools and Techniques of Biotechnology

Q9

What is gram positive?

Q10

What is a spectrophotometer?

A9

A bacterial cell that stains purple (or blue) after Gram staining

A10

An instrument that measures the amount of light (of a known wavelength) absorbed by a sample

Q11

What can a spectrophotometer be used for?

Q12

What is pH?

A11

♦ **Determine the concentration of a solution because amount of absorption is proportional to concentration**

♦ **Identify a molecule**

♦ **Determine change in samples over time**

A12

The level of acid or base in a solution

Q13

What is a pH meter?

Q14

What is the range of pH values?

A13

An instrument that measures the pH of a solution

A14

0-14

pH=0 means highest level of acidity

pH=14 means highest level of basicity

pH=7 means neutral such as water

Q15

What is the recombinant DNA technique?

Q16

What are the main steps involved in a recombinant DNA technique to produce protein?

A15

The technique used to cut and recombine DNA molecules

A16

1. **Identify, and isolate (cut) or produce a copy of the desired DNA sequence that has the code for producing the desired protein.**

2. **Insert this DNA sequence into the host cell such as a bacterial cell.**

3. **Induce the host cell to produce proteins according to the instructions in the DNA sequence.**

4. **Collect and purify the newly produced protein molecules.**

Q17

What is DNA Sequencing?

Q18

List some DNA sequencing techniques.

A17

The process of determining the order of nucleotides (A, G, C, T) in a DNA fragment

A18

- ♦ **Maxam-Gilbert sequencing**

- ♦ **Sanger technique**

- ♦ **High throughput sequencing methods**

Q19

What is Maxam-Gilbert sequencing?

Q20

What is Sanger technique?

A19

A DNA sequencing method, developed in 1976-77 by Allan Maxam and Walter Gilbert, that is based on chemical modification of DNA

A20

The most popular DNA sequencing technique, developed by Fredrick Sanger et. al. in 1975, that is based on the DNA chain termination

Q21

What are high throughput sequencing methods?

Q22

What is chromatography?

A21

A set of DNA sequencing methods that are designed to speed up the sequencing process by using techniques such as parallel sequencing

A22

A set of techniques used to separate components of a mixture. The components to be separated are distributed between two phases: stationary phase and mobile phase that allows motion in a specific direction.

Q23

What is column chromatography?

Q24

What is HPLC?

A23

A chromatographic technique in which the stationary bed is inside a tube, called column

A24

High performance liquid chromatography; a column chromatography that uses metal columns to withstand high pressure. It is often used to identify and quantify molecules.

Q25

What are some of the tools to measure volumes in a biotechnology lab?

Q26

How precisely can you measure mass in a biotechnology lab?

A25

- **Graduated cylinder.** 10 mL to 2L

- **Pipet.** 0.1 mL to 50 mL

- **Micropipet.** 0.5 µL to 1 mL

A26

Most analytical balances with electronic display can measure mass down to milligrams.

Q27

What is PCR?

Q28

What is sterilization?

A27

Polymerase chain reaction; a technique used to make copies of a DNA fragment with an exponentially amplified speed

A28

A process that eliminates (e.g. kills) contaminating agents such as bacteria, fungi, and viruses from anything such as equipment, food, or biological culture medium

Q29

How is sterilization achieved?

Q30

What is a sterile technique?

A29

By applying chemicals, filtration, heat, or high pressure

A30

The set of practices to transfer content from one container to another without contaminating it

Q31

What is an autoclave?

Q32

This is an analytical technique to separate molecules based on their electric charge, size, or both:

A31

A heavy vessel used to achieve sterilization through heat and pressure

A32

Electrophoresis

Q33

What is western blot?

Q34

The vessel in which the biosynthetic operations occur:

A33

A process that uses gel electrophoresis to detect a specific protein in a sample

A34

Bioreactor

Q35

Chemicals captured from living cells and used as reagents in production processes are called:

Q36

True or false: If a piece of equipment is clean, it means it's sterilized.

A35

Bioreagents

A36

False; an object may look clean even when it's not sterilized.

   Tools and Techniques of Biotechnology

Q1

What is a plant?

Q2

The transfer of male gametes in a plant flower, the pollen, to its female part, the pistil, is called:

A1

A plant is a multicellular eukaryote that creates organic molecules through photosynthesis. In other words, plants produce their own food through photosynthesis.

A2

Pollination

Q3

This is the process of propagating plants (or animals for that matter) through sexual reproduction by pre-determined specific parents:

Q4

During breeding, the cell division called meiosis produces sperm and egg cells called:

A3

Breeding

A4

Gametes

Q5

This is the process in which each of two parent cells contributes a set of chromosomes carried by the gametes to produce offspring:

Q6

A plant (or animal) in its initial stage of development:

A5

Sexual reproduction

A6

Embryo

Q7

The cells that have not yet differentiated themselves into specific functionalities, but have the potential to differentiate (or specialize) into any functionality are called:

Q8

Stem cells existing in adult tissues are called adult stem cells, whereas stem cells derived from embryos are called:

A7

Stem cells

A8

Embryonic stem cells

Q9

What is tissue culture?

Q10

This is the mass of undifferentiated plant cells developed during the growth of tissue culture:

A9

The process of growing plant (or animal) cells in a sterile medium that contains the nutrients required for the growth

A10

Callus

Q11

These cells have two sets of chromosomes, called homologous chromosomes, usually one from each parent:

Q12

True or false: Plants (and animals) are diploid organisms.

A11

Diploid cells

A12

True

Q13

What is an allele?

Q14

What is genetic cross?

A13

A member of a pair or a series of genes that occupy a specific position on a specific chromosome. Some alleles are dominant, whereas others are recessive.

A14

A process to predict the traits of the offspring

Q15

What is a Punnett square?

Q16

Consider a male and female both with genotypes Bb, where B is a dominant allele and b is a recessive allele. Draw the Punnett square for the genotypes of their offspring.

A15

A diagram used by biologists to determine the probability of the traits of an offspring given the genotype (genetic constitution) of the parents

A16

Male alleles (B and b) combining with female alleles (B and b) to form different genotypes for the offspring:

	Male B	Male b
Female B	BB	Bb
Female b	Bb	bb

Probability for BB: 25%

Probability for bb: 25%

Probability for Bb: 50%

Q17

This is the technique in which pollen is taken from one plant and is used for fertilization in another plant:

Q18

What is a foreign (or an alien) gene?

A17

Crossbreeding

A18

The gene in an organism that has been transported into it from another organism. For example, some varieties of corn in USA have genes inserted into them from certain bacteria or fungi.

Q19

The crops (food) with foreign genes, called transgenes, are known as:

Q20

Crops are made insect resistant by using THIS bacteria because it produces protein that kills the insects:

A19

Genetically modified (GM) crops (foods)

A20

Bt; Bacillus thuringiensis

Q21

The resistance of GM crops to viruses is called:

Q22

True or false: Herbicide tolerance is one of the major areas of genetic engineering of crops.

A21

Pathogen resistance

A22

True

Q23

True or false: GM food is usually less nutrient.

Q24

True-false: Genetical engineering of farm animals causes increased productivity of animal-based food products.

A23

False. Mostly, the GM crops are nutritionally enhanced crops. Golden rice is an example.

A24

True

Q25

A technique used to produce identical organisms through asexual reproduction:

Q26

True or false: Embryonic stem cells were used in the first successful cloning that produced Dolly the sheep.

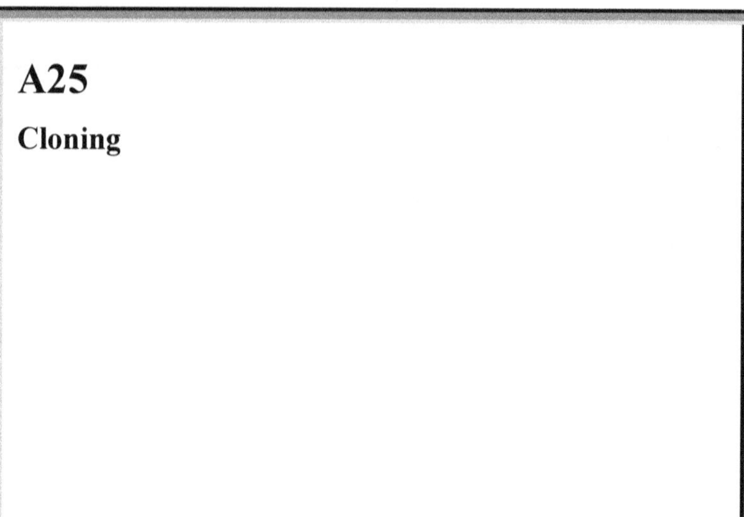

A25

Cloning

A26

False. Dolly the sheep cloning was derived from adult cells.

Q27

This is the practice of growing plants in a soil-less but water-based medium, that is, the mineral nutrient solution:

Q28

In a mature or developing organism, the line (i.e. sequence) of cells such as sex cells that hold the genetic material that can be passed on to the offspring is called:

A27

Hydroponics

A28

Germline

Q29

Cells that are not in the germline but make the body of an organism are called:

Q30

A female reproductive cell (gamete) is called:

A29

Somatic cells

A30

Ovum; plural ova

Q31

What is SCNT?

Q32

Absence of cleft in chin (C) is a dominant gene, whereas presence of cleft in chin (c) is a recessive gene. Male alleles (c and c) from a parent with cleft in chin combine with female alleles (C and c) from parent with no cleft in chin. What is the probability that the offspring will have cleft in chin?

A31

Somatic cell nuclear transfer; a technique used to create an ovum with a donor nucleus; the nucleus of a fertilized egg is replaced with the nucleus from a somatic cell. The cell behaves like an embryonic stem cell, but actually has the genetic material derived from an adult cell.

A32

Male alleles (C and C) combining with female alleles (C and c) to form different genotypes for the offspring:

	Male c	Male c
Female C	Cc	Cc
Female c	cc	cc

Probability for cleft in chin, cc: 50%

Probability for no cleft in chin Cc + CC: 50%

Q1

True or false: DNA of all organisms is composed of the same physical and chemical components.

Q2

The complete set of DNA of an organism is called:

A1

True

A2

Genome

 Biotechnology of DNA

Q3

DNA in the human genome is arranged into how many distinct chromosomes?

Q4

True or false: All human cells except the mature red blood cells contain a complete genome.

A3

24; 22 non-sexual, and 2 sexual (X and Y)

A4

True

Q5

How many chromosomes does a human (somatic) cell has?

Q6

What is a chromosome?

A5

23 chromosome pairs: One member of each pair (1 through 22) from each parent, plus an X chromosome from the female parent and an X or Y chromosome from the male parent. This adds up to a total of 46 chromosomes.

A6

An organized structure of DNA that contains genes and some proteins

Q7

What are genes?

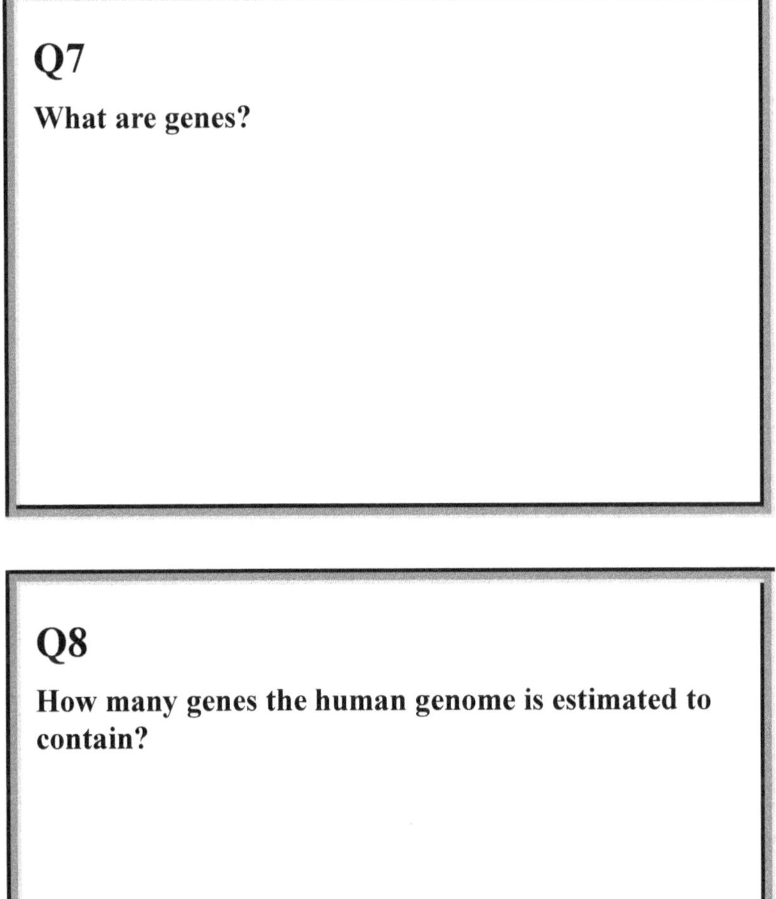

Q8

How many genes the human genome is estimated to contain?

A7

Basic functional and physical units of heredity that contain instructions on how to make proteins. These instructions are in terms of specific sequences of bases in a gene.

A8

20,000 – 25,000

Q9

A chromosome molecule contains about how many base pairs?

Q10

The human genome contains about how many DNA base pairs?

A9

About 50 million to 250 million

A10

Three billion

150 million base pairs per chromosome x 23 chromosomes

Q11

True or false: The genes that code for proteins only make about 2% of the human genome.

Q12

For over 50% of the human genome, no function has yet been determined or identified. This portion of the genome is called:

A11

True. The remainder of genome (about 98%) consists of non-coding regions, which provide functionalities such as chromosomal structural integrity, and regulating the production of protein: where, when, and in what quantity.

A12

Junk DNA

Q13

The 22 non-sexual pairs of chromosomes in the human genome are called:

Q14

True or false: A human body is estimated to typically consists of 20 trillion cells, all of which originate from a single fertilized egg cell by means of cell division which includes DNA replication.

A13

Homologous pairs

A14

True

Q15

What is a DNA Probe?

Q16

The combination of a natural DNA strand and a probe strand is called:

A15

The instrument (or system) used to reveal the base sequence of an existing DNA. It consists of a complementary DNA strand that will detect the base DNA strand because both base and complementary strands will be attracted to each other. For example, a base sequence A-C-T-G-G will be detected by the complementary sequence T-G-A-C-C.

A16

Hybrid

Q17

The process of binding the nucleic acids of the complementary DNA strand to those of the base DNA strand is called:

Q18

Before it could be probed, the sample of a natural DNA is heated to obtain the single strands. This process is called:

A17

Hybridization

A18

Denaturation

Q19

DNA probe is also called a:

Q20

For visualization and analysis, the DNA fragments on a gel are transferred to an electrically charged membrane called blot. This process is called:

A19

Nuclear probe

A20

Southern blotting

Q21

These are the enzymes used to build large molecules, called polymers, from smaller molecules, called monomers:

Q22

By running down the template strand, a polymerase builds a complementary DNA strand. This polymerase is called a:

A21

Polymerase

A22

DNA polymerase

Q23

What is a template DNA?

Q24

What are the sources of A, C, G, and T used to synthesize a new DNA strand?

A23

The DNA strand by reading which a new (complementary) DNA strand is synthesized

---

A24

dATP; deoxyadenosine triphosphate; source for adenine (A).

dCTP; deoxycytidine triphosphate; source for cytosine (C).

dGTP; deoxyguanosine triphosphate; source for guanine (G).

dTTP; deoxthymidine triphosphate; source for thymine (T).

Q25

True or false: DNA replication (synthesis) can be performed in the lab.

Q26

What is PAGE?

A25

True

A26

Polyacrylamide gel electrophoresis; a technique used to separate protein and DNA molecules through electrophoresis on vertical gels.

www.ingramcontent.com/pod-product-compliance
Lightning Source LLC
Chambersburg PA
CBHW071550030726
47593CB00001BA/104